Beating Back Pain Through Diet

By Lynne D M Noble

Copyright 2024 Lynne D M Noble

Independently published

Contents

Preface

When I was researching for this book on back pain. I came across this on the NHS website:[1]

Back pain is very common and normally improves within weeks or months.

Pain in the lower back (lumbago) is particularly common, although it can be felt anywhere along the spine – from the neck down to the hips.

In most cases the pain isn't caused by anything serious and will usually get better over time.

There are things you can do to help relieve it. However, the pain can last a long time or keep coming back.

Now you may be wondering what point I am trying to make. After all, the above statement is merely reflecting the truth, isn't it? Well, back pain is debilitating. It is the cause of hours and hours of misery and lost working days and life

---

[1] https://www.nhs.uk/conditions/back-pain/

quality. Yet we seem to think that it is acceptable that an improvement is unlikely for weeks or months. Further, even if we can do something about it the pain can still last for a long time and/or keep coming back.

This isn't really acceptable when the level of pain can climb off the scale and painkillers, like ibuprofen and paracetamol appear to barely touch it. In some cases, these analgesics fail to touch the pain at all. There is a reason for that as we shall see in the book, later.

Many GP's do not refer to a physiotherapist for six weeks. They prefer a wait and see approach.

They may advise on keeping active but when every little movement is agonising, then there is little motivation to keep going. Bed seems a good idea but that just gives you time to think about the pain. Trying to roll over in bed is torture. You are dependent for the first time in your life for someone to put your shoes and socks on.

If you are given medication which is stronger than paracetamol or ibuprofen, then it is likely to make you even less motivated as it will cause a hungover brain fog effect. In addition, it will probably make you constipated for the first time in your life. Does it really have to be like this?

Back pain really isn't any fun and it should be treated with a little more understanding and compassion.

This book shows you what is likely to go wrong in back pain and what you can do about it. It looks at common back complaints such as sciatica and lumbago, among others, helping you to understand the underlying problems and, more importantly, showing you what you can do to shorten the recovery time as well as reduce the pain.

It is generally the case that the wrong type of painkiller is given so it is not surprising that medication does not work but we will look at that in more detail. It is also true that inflammatory pain can occur alongside neuropathic pain in which case treatment for both needs to be considered. Then there is the difference between acute inflammatory and chronic inflammatory pain which once recognised, in the case of the latter, needs further investigation. While acute inflammation is due to infection or injury, it should eventually resolve; chronic pain is pathological and is never something that should be put up with due to 'ageing' or something similar. The body is designed to heal itself so if it doesn't then it is highly likely that a nutritional deficiency has some part to play.

It helps to understand the vertebrae when we are looking at the concept of back pain so that is where we shall begin.

The spine and vertebrae

The spine is a marvellous structure designed to protect and allow movement.

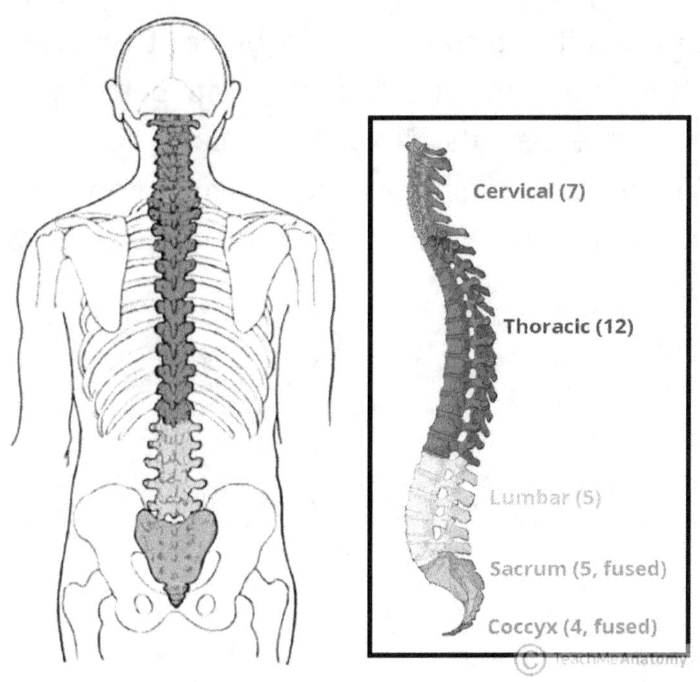

2

It consists of 33 vertebrae of which seven are the cervical vertebrae, 12 make up the thoracic

---

2 https://teachmeanatomy.info/back/bones/vertebral-column/

section, 5 make up the lumbar area, the fused sacrum consists of five and finally the coccyx consists of 4 fused vertebrae.

Although the primary function of the vertebrae is a protective one as the spinal cord runs through it, it also helps to provide structure and attachment for the pectoral and pelvic girdles and muscles. Its flexibility occurs due to the ligaments and spinal discs. This allows us to bend forwards and backwards and twist and turn.

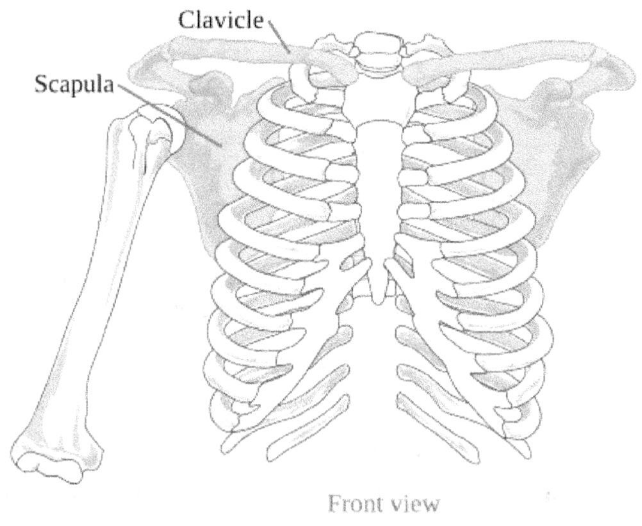

Front view

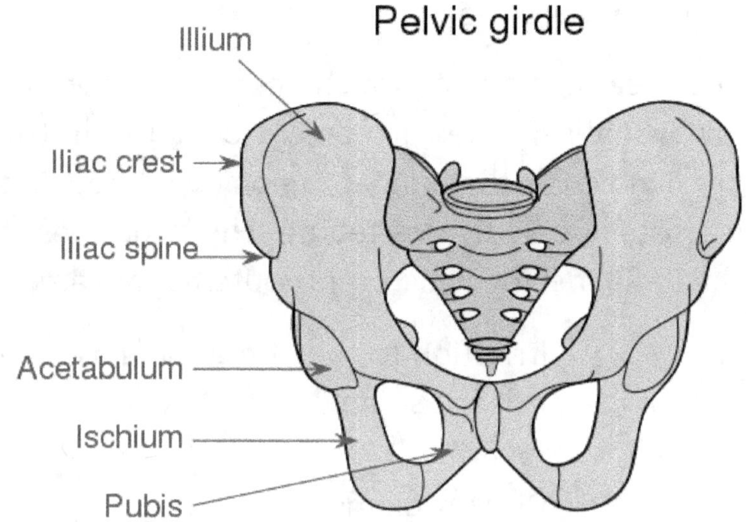

The pelvic girdle

The spinal cord is the main pathway for information between the brain and peripheral nervous system. It is a huge cord which looks rather like a bunch of telephone wires all bundled together. These exit the vertebrae at intervals and enter the peripheral nervous system.

The peripheral nervous system consists of the nerves outside the brain and spinal cord.

The area of the back which appears to be most problematical when it comes to injury, is the area known as the lumbar region even though it consists of only five vertebrae. The structures in the lumbar spine which contribute to pain are:

- Irritation to the nerve roots as they exit the spine
- Arthritis
- Disc problems
- Problems with bones
- Problems with muscles

It is not unusual to find one problem will set another off a bit like a stack of dominoes which set off a chain reaction. For example, a sudden jerk can damage a disc which can then protrude and irritate a nerve ending.

Pain can be classified as either axial pain or radicular pain. Axial back pain is pain which remains in the spine while radicular pain is pain which radiates down the legs as can be felt in sciatica.

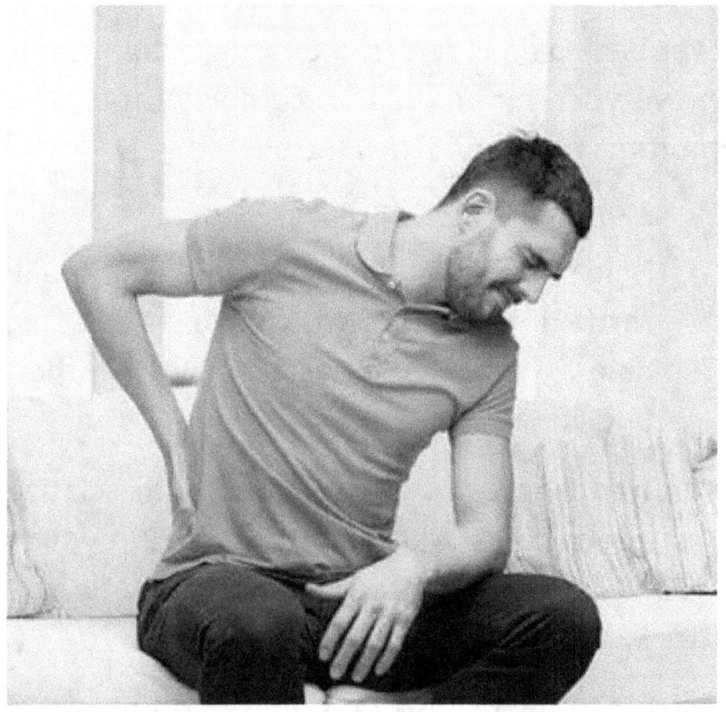

Sciatica starts in the spine where injury compresses the nerve causing debilitating radicular pain. It is the most common manifestation of irritation to the nerve root.

Common back pain problems

Lower back pain is referred to as lumbago and it is a very common health complaint but the symptoms can vary. They include:

- Acute pain
- Mild discomfort which may eventually settle into a pattern known as chronic pain – that is, it lasts for more than twelve weeks.

Often lumbago can be associated with sciatica which tends to be a quite intense 'ache' which travels down from the lower back into the buttock, leg and eventually foot.

Sciatica can also cause numbness and pins and needles in the affected leg. Sciatica is very painful and most people find the tasks of daily living just about impossible. In spite of this, most back pain is referred to as 'non-specific' in that it does not appear to be related to any specific dysfunction.

Specific dysfunction can be:

- Disc related
- Facet joint related
- Muscular
- Pelvic or sacral dysfunction

With any back pain the danger signs are:

- Drop foot or an altered gait pattern
- Urinary retention
- Saddle anaesthesia – where there is numbness around the saddle area
- Bilateral pins and needles
- Loss of leg strength

If any of the above occur, then you should seek an immediate referral to the GP.

Lumbago can sometimes be caused by a herniated disc more commonly known as a slipped disc. Some slipped discs do not appear to cause problems for people but, for others, they cause terrible and intractable pain. Other common reasons for lumbago are osteoporosis and osteoarthritis. We shall look at these in more detail later.

Under the umbrella term of lumbago, we shall look at:

- Sciatica
- Osteoporosis
- Osteoarthritis

We will look at them separately in order to ascertain what is causing the pain and what we can do about it.

Sciatica

When I was working in orthopaedics, it was not uncommon to find rows of patients lying on their back attached to traction. The idea behind this was to separate – slightly - the discs which were causing pressure on the nerves in the hope that it would relieve the pain.

I cannot actually recall this treatment working any more quickly than it would take to recover naturally. Since the patients were often flat on their backs for weeks, the pain and inflammation probably died a natural death as do many inflammatory states, eventually.

The sciatic nerve is the longest nerve in the body and when pressure or damage occurs then the debilitating pain will start. A timely response to the initial injury or start of sciatic pain can help to reduce the severity and duration of this disabling condition.

Treatment of sciatic pain

- Apply ice packs for the first three days as this will help to reduce inflammation. After three days alternate cold and heat packs. The cold pack will continue to reduce the inflammation and the heat packs will draw blood to the area to take away toxins. Heat will also help to reduce spasm. Muscle spasms are very painful.

- Some people will take paracetamol and ibuprofen as prescribed on the packet. Both are generally taken together as paracetamol works in the central nervous system and ibuprofen works in the peripheral nervous system. Taking painkillers with strong coffee will also help reduce the pain. Caffeine helps painkillers to enter the bloodstream quickly and efficiently. Caffeine is sometimes added to painkillers because of it pain alleviating effects. Coffee also contains powerful antioxidants which help to neutralise inflammation.

However, nutritional medicine is far superior to paracetamol and ibuprofen. The end product of metabolism of paracetamol is phenacetin which was removed from the market decades ago as it was linked to dementia.

Ibuprofen is high risk for ulcers in the gastrointestinal tract in the same way as aspirin is. It is often the case that, in using prescription, or over the counter medications, to treat one condition, that is induces others.

Far better is to use some very natural nutrients and products. Vitamin C has anti-inflammatory properties in high enough doses known as 'therapeutic' doses.

People are wary of 'therapeutic doses' which are far higher than the recommended daily intake. However, the recommended daily intake of vitamin C is the very minimum needed to prevent scurvy. It does not take into account that much higher doses are required, on a daily basis, to maintain optimum health in other parts of the body. Indeed, when sciatica does occur then at least 2g (2000mg) of vitamin C daily is needed.

Adding in 300mg of magnesium will enhance the effect of vitamin C.

Liniment rub:

In order to alleviate the pain and reduce inflammation externally, a simple liniment rub can be made. This consists of:

One tablespoon full of DMSO (I use 99%) and

One teaspoonful of camphor oil

Mix together well and rub into the affected part.

This and the vitamin C with magnesium can deal with sciatic pain within 24 hours or less rather than the 6 weeks, GP's allow before sending you to see a physiotherapist.

I will talk more of DMSO later in the book.

Some people also find it helpful to take antihistamines:

- **In the first few days, an antihistamine may be taken. This may sound peculiar but following any injury, an inflammatory mediator called histamine helps to widen blood vessels and make them leaky. This extra fluid presses on nerves and irritates them further.**

However, antihistamines have negative side effects. In small doses for a few days only, they are acceptable but vitamin C is able to quell the release of histamine and do not have the side effects of antihistamines which are:

Weight gain

Somnolence

Constipation

Prolonged use is also linked with dementia

Muscle spasm with sciatica causing pain

It is quite likely that the muscles will go into spasm. Spasms cause more pain than the original injury. Any movement tends to send the muscles into spasm until it unfortunately becomes the 'default' mode.

The muscle knot or spasm can be quite pronounced. It can feel rigid and unyielding held in this unnatural position. It is meant to be a position which protects the original injury but it often feels much worse and often the body does not know when to let go of its protective stance and return back to normal.

Massages help but they don't tend to get to the centre of the spasm. Pressing a finger or a knuckle into the centre of the spasm - which is initially exquisitely painful - and holding it until the pain dissolves - is a tried and tested remedy.

I normally push a finger or rubber tip of a pencil, in the middle of a spasm and work outwards until I can feel all the spasm has dissipated. This may need doing a few times but it is one of the most effective pain relievers that I know.

Some soreness may remain due to the lactic acid build up that occurs when muscles have knotted but it is nothing compared to acute sciatic pain. Thankfully, the soreness due to lactic acid soon goes.

Lactic acid is produced in your muscles and builds up during intense exercise. It is released into the muscles when the muscles have used up their normal energy stores but still need further energy.

Lactic acid is, in effect, a temporary energy source but if too much builds up, the familiar 'burning' sensations found in muscles after intense exercise can be felt.

  When your muscles have gone into spasm they also produce lactic acid which can cause pain and soreness.

During normal exercise, the soreness is only temporary but when the muscles have tightened for a long time during a spasm, the lactic acid continues to build up.

As people get older, their fingers and knuckles are not up to this sort of pressure. The 'emergency' kit to replace fingers is a lip salve or lipstick container.

I first discovered the benefits of this piece of equipment when I suffered from piriformis syndrome. This is a condition which is extremely painful. Piriformis syndrome occurs on the outer thigh.

In order to take the piriformis, muscle out of spasm, the attending physiotherapist normally inserts their elbow into the part of the thigh where this tiny, but deep, muscle is.

Of course, unless we are contortionists, we cannot do this. However, as we all know necessity breeds invention and I never travel without a lip salve container now. It is an invaluable piece of equipment when it comes to taking muscular spasms out of default mode.

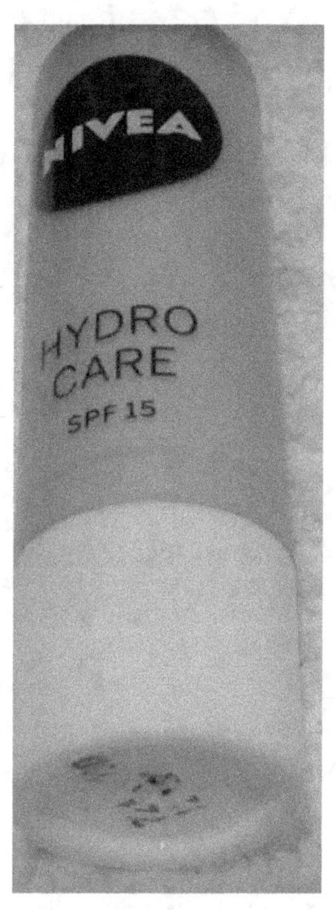

I have found that this little piece of equipment is far more effective than the anti-spasmodic medication that is often prescribed which includes medications such as diazepam or baclofen.

Burning muscles are not only due to too much lactic acid but also to too little oxygen. Breathing deeply will help to correct the latter.

Some athletes have used sodium bicarbonate (baking soda) mixed with water to act as a buffer which raises the pH of the body temporarily and helps remove lactic acid. However, sodium bicarbonate can:

- Raise blood pressure due to its sodium content
- Belching
- Diarrhoea

Creative monohydrate can be used as a substitute for sodium bicarbonate.

Leucine, an essential amino acid, also helps improve muscle recovery after exercise.

Magnesium is a marvellous mineral which has antispasmodic properties. It is a calming mineral which helps to reduce pain and it is essential for proper muscle function.

300mg daily should suffice although some people swear by magnesium oil which can be rubbed into the sore places.

To help magnesium penetrate more deeply mix it with a little DMSO.

Phenylalanine is an amino acid which can be used as an adjunctive pain reliever. It can also be taken alone. It helps to raise pain thresholds and increase tolerance to pain. It works by blocking enzymes that break down two of the body's pain relieving substances – encephalin and endorphins.

An encephalin is a small protein molecule which helps regulate pain in the body. They bind to the body's opioid receptors.

Opioid receptors can be found in the brain. Opioids made in the body attach to these receptors and help block pain as well as having an anti-depressant effect.

It can be understood that it would be helpful to block enzymes which would break these natural pain relievers down. Phenylalanine does just that.

Phenylalanine acts on endorphins in a similar way to that of encephalin.

Although it is possible to supplement phenylalanine – and many people do supplement, phenylalanine is found in a wide range of foods which include:

All animal proteins such as

Fish

Meat

Eggs

Dairy

Vegetable based proteins such as:

Nuts

Beans

Tofu

And it is found in non-protein foods such as:

Carbonated drinks and foods containing aspartame

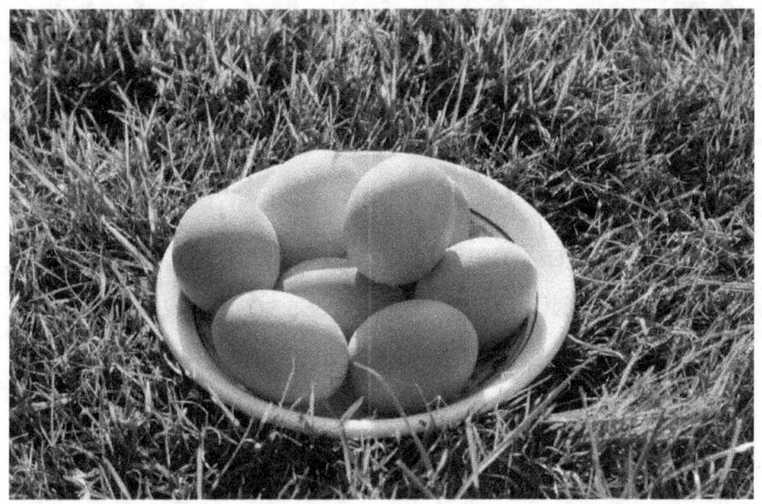

Eggs: a good source of phenylalanine

The role of glycine

It would be remiss of me if I did not add glycine as one of the mainstays of the back sufferer's emergency kit. Glycine can relieve intractable back pain in less than a day and continue to employ its anti-inflammatory and analgesic properties if it is taken on a daily basis in sufficient amounts.

There is no reason why this should not be so. Glycine is the smallest amino acid of the twenty amino acids. Only nine are essential; glycine is a non- essential amino acid so it is capable of being synthesised by the body when needed.

That's the official story but….

 Our current diets do not support the synthesis of enough glycine to support the healthy bones, muscle tissue, ligaments, tendons and cartilage (which cushion the spinal discs) required for a pain free back.

Let's look at some of the actions of this marvellous building block of connective tissue.

Glycine is an inhibitory amino acid which means that it helps to calm your brain down. This also reduces the sensation of pain. It also helps to absorb calcium which is good news for those with osteoarthritis and osteoporosis.

Glycine acts directly on cells which are involved in the inflammatory process. It suppresses free radicals which are highly reactive molecules that go around – like an out of control pinball – damaging cells which get in its way. Glycine also suppresses inflammatory cytokines.

Inflammatory cytokines are molecules which are secreted from immune cells like macrophages. They help promote inflammation. Of course, it is the inflammatory processes which cause the pain.

Fructose is a type of sugar commonly found in fruit. It has the ability to raise inflammation through a cell signalling molecule called Tumour Necrosis Factor (TNF). Glycine has the ability to block this process and further block another molecule called interleukin 6 which is also involved in the inflammatory process.

However, while our first thought after a back injury is to alleviate the pain, our next thoughts must turn to helping build strong connective tissue – in all its forms – in order to try and prevent back injury from happening again.

This is where glycine comes into its own as it is the major building block of the protein collagen which is found in all connective tissue.

This means that it has amazing benefits not just for lumbago but also osteoarthritis and osteoporosis which we will look at in a short while.

Where can glycine be found? Glycine is normally found in many of the foods that we don't eat nowadays. These include:

- Bone broths
- Chicken skin
- Pork scratchings
- Pigs ears
- Tripe
- Organ meats

to name but a few.

In WW1 and WW2 and the immediate post war years, these foods were eaten on a regular basis. Food was scarce and so nothing was wasted. Fish heads were kept to one side to make fish head soup. Chicken bones were stewed slowly until they yielded a clear broth full of goodness. What they all had in common was a protein called gelatine which is the cooked form of collagen.

Gelatine contains 23% of glycine. It plumps up connective tissue making it strong – and in the case of tendons, ligaments and skin – flexible. Bones and muscles are made stronger.

As age progresses, sarcopenia can occur. Sarcopenia is age-related muscle wasting. As muscles waste then joints are not held as strongly as they used to be; they are not up to the job that they were designed to do.

 You don't get many children with the sort of back problems that adults suffer from, increasingly as they get older. I don't know of any child with lumbago. Yes, there are genetic predispositions to certain joint and back problems but, on the whole, these injuries are not due to muscle wasting.

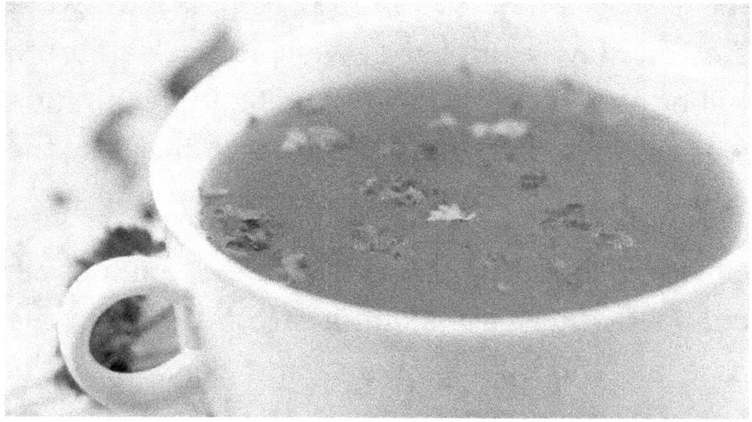

Bone broth; the perfect nutritional medicine for joint and back problems and sarcopenia

You can see that age related muscle loss has a lot to answer for although the loss of flexibility, which is also addressed by glycine, cannot be discounted.

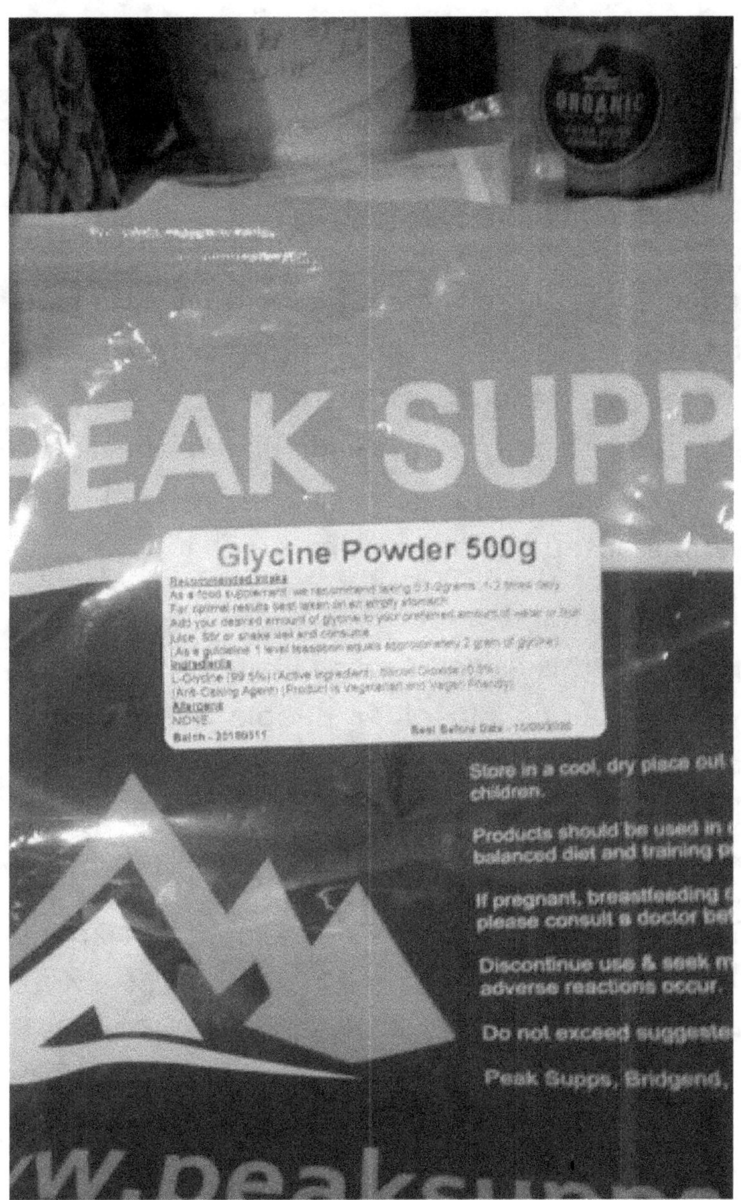
PEAK SUPP
Glycine Powder 500g
Recommended Usage
As a food supplement, we recommend taking 5-3 grams, 1-2 times daily.
For optimal results best taken on an empty stomach.
Add your desired amount of glycine to your prepared amount of water or fruit
juice. Stir or shake well and consume.
(As a guideline, 1 level teaspoon equals approximately 2 gram of glycine)
Ingredients
L-Glycine (99.5%) (Active Ingredient), Silicon Dioxide (0.5%)
(Anti-Caking Agent) (Product is vegetarian and Vegan Friendly)
Allergens
NONE
Batch - 20180511
Best Before Date - 10/09/2020
Store in a cool, dry place out
children.
Products should be used in
balanced diet and training p
If pregnant, breastfeeding
please consult a doctor bef
Discontinue use & seek m
adverse reactions occur.
Do not exceed suggeste
Peak Supps, Bridgend,
w.peaksu

Normally, the task of building up muscle, is the domain of another amino acid called leucine.

Leucine is an essential amino acid which means that we must get it from dietary sources since our bodies cannot synthesise it. It is called a Branched Chain Amino Acid (BCAA) and is the most abundant in muscle tissue. It is found in all animal sources of protein.

Leucine stimulates protein synthesis and muscle tissue but this effect is more likely to be seen in younger people. In older people or in people who have muscle wasting diseases, glycine is the amino acid which helps the synthesis of lean muscle tissue.

Glycine combined with L- theanine (an amino acid found in tea) helps the recovery of tendonitis. Further, as it has oestrogen like effects, it helps to protect bones.

Glycine can be made from glutamic acid. Glutamic acid is an amino acid which is found in:

- All types of meat
- Dairy
- Eggs
- Fish

The main vegetarian source of glutamic acid is wheat. Pasta and bread form the staple diets of many and should provide all the glycine that we need but, it appears, that many individuals who are on vegan or vegetarian diets may be low in glycine.

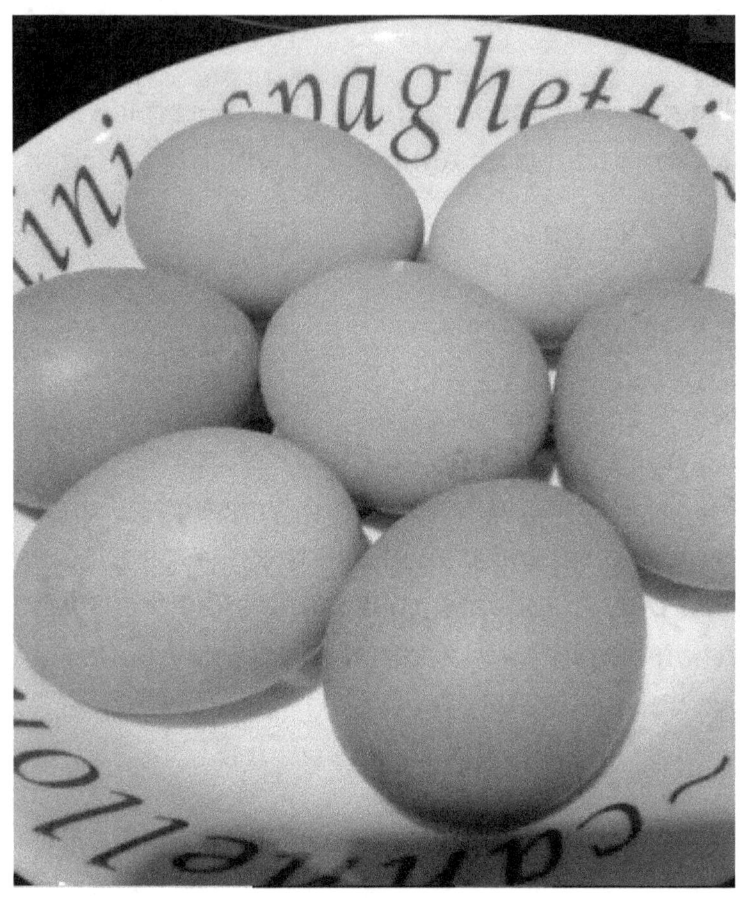

Eggs and pasta are full of glutamic acid which is a precursor to glycine.

Glycine is a white crystalline, sweet tasting substance. It resembles sugar and, as such, is good for sprinkling on cereals and stirring into drinks if you wish to sweeten them.'

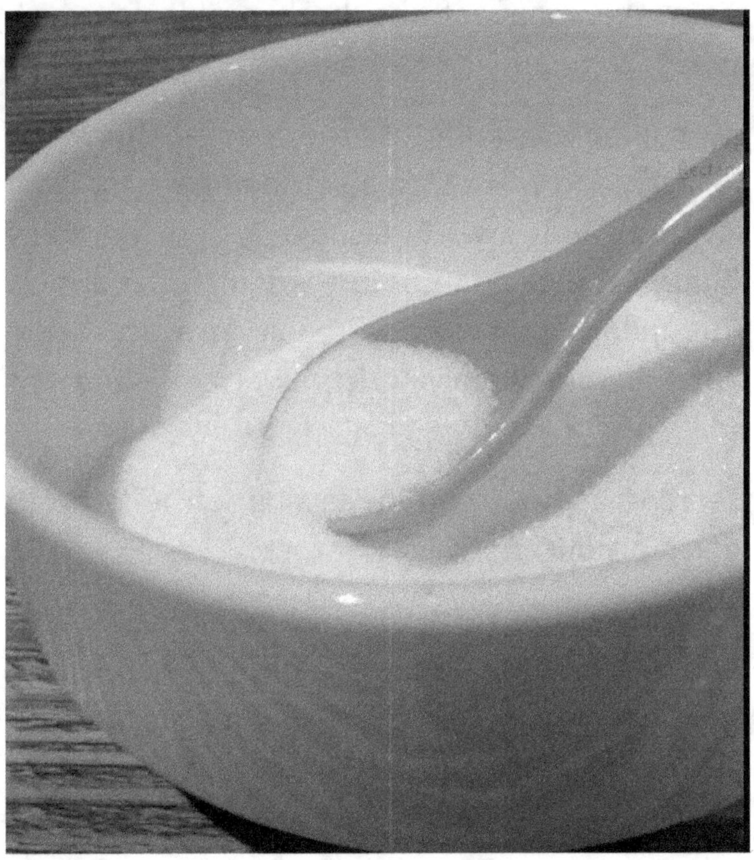

Glycine is a sweet crystalline substance resembling sugar.

I would always recommend that an increase in collagen forming amino acids - especially glycine – is incorporated into the diet once the middle twenties are reached. Following this guideline may save many of the back problems which appear to be rife in older age.

Of course, gelatine is the cooked form of collagen and is used as a setting agent for both savoury and sweet dishes. You normally 'bloom' the gelatine before adding it to dishes. This means that you soften it in a little cold water before dissolving it in warmer – but not boiling – liquid.

Gelatine can be seen in 'setting' of bone broth which produces a jelly like stock.

It is also the substance of wine gums and gummy bears. If you are laid up in bed with a bad back, ask for wine gums instead of chocolate!

Boron is a trace element which is required in the body in tiny amounts but any deficiency will have serious side effects. These include:

- Neural malfunction
- Osteoporosis
- Arthritis
- Hormone imbalance
- Hyperthyroidism
- Abnormal metabolism of calcium

A number of studies in both controlled animal and human studies have provided evidence for the use of boron as a safe and effective treatment for osteoarthritis. These studies have shown that in areas where boron intake is greater than, or equal to one milligram daily, the estimated incidence of arthritis ranges from 20 -70%. In areas where boron intake is usually 3mg to 10mg daily, the estimated incidence of arthritis ranges from 0-10% which is significantly lower.

The boron concentration was found to be lower in the femur heads, bones and synovial fluid of patients with osteoarthritis compared with individuals who did not have osteoarthritis.

Boron has also been found to downregulate enzymes involved in the inflammatory response.

In the severe OA group, average pain reduction was 47.9% at 4 weeks and 64.5% at 8 weeks.

In the first 4 weeks, 40% of subjects with severe OA reduced or eliminated their analgesic use (ibuprofen).

By week 8, 75% had quit using their NSAID medication (ibuprofen. Joint rigidity disappeared in one half of the severe OA patients in the first 4 weeks.

In the remaining one-half of the severe OA, joint rigidity decreased significantly, an average rigidity reduction of 50% of severe OA subjects at 4 weeks and in 62.5% at 8 weeks.

More recently, calcium fructoborate 110mg which provides approximately 3mg of boron 2X daily or 6mg daily, was shown to improve knee discomfort within the first 14 days of treatment.

There is an upper limit (UL) of 20mg daily and effects of boron do not appear to occur until a minimum of 3mg daily is taken.

Good sources of boron per 100g are:

- Raisins 4.51mg
- Almonds 2.82mg
- Hazelnuts 77mg
- Dried apricots 2.11mg
- Peanut butter 1.92mg
- Brazil nuts 1.72mg
- Walnuts 1.63mg
- Red kidney beans 1.4mg
- Prunes 1.18mg
- Cashew nuts (raw) 1.15mg
- Dates 1.08mg
- Chickpeas 0.71mg
- Lentils 0.74mg
- Peaches 0.52mg

Although another good sources of boron are brazil nuts, these contain selenium which is toxic if more than two are eaten daily. Therefore, it is not recommended that you eat more than two brazil nuts daily.

Our plan of action for generalised back pain is now summarised below.

Treatment	Application
cold packs	Days 1-3
hot and cold packs	From day 3 until pain/injury is resolved
phenylalanine	Follow instructions on the packet
Magnesium and vitamin C	400mg 2g
lip salve container and leucine (if lactic acid build up)	For muscle spasms
glycine	2-4 teaspoons daily
antihistamine	Take the first as soon as the injury occurs
Increase gelatin intake DMSO and camphor liniment	Animal skin/bones although there is a vegetarian version

Phenylalanine and glycine are both obtainable from health foods shops and online, as is leucine, in cases of muscle soreness due to lactic acid build up.

Prostaglandins which contribute to pain along with histamine are normally dealt with by the use of an anti-inflammatory like ibuprofen. Some people develop allergies to NSAIDS like ibuprofen.

People who are on medication such as the disease modifying drugs (DMARD's) are advised against taking anti-inflammatories.

A good, natural anti-inflammatory which help reduce the pain producing prostaglandins is fresh ginger.

Bradykinin is another substance which induces pain after injury. Fresh pineapple effectively combats the effects of bradykinin.

Bradykinin is linked with conditions such as:

Lesions brought about by the immune system

Sepsis and

Acute lung infection/injury

Using this knowledge, we can see that some freshly grated ginger into fresh pineapple sweetened with glycine to taste will assist the treatment programme for back pain.

Enzymes in pineapple effectively address the inflammation caused by bradykinin

Osteoporosis and Osteoarthritis

When I was very young, I saw many elderly – and not so elderly – people stooped over in a very unnatural fashion. Indeed, my maternal grandmother had the typical hunchback of what I now know to be osteoporosis.

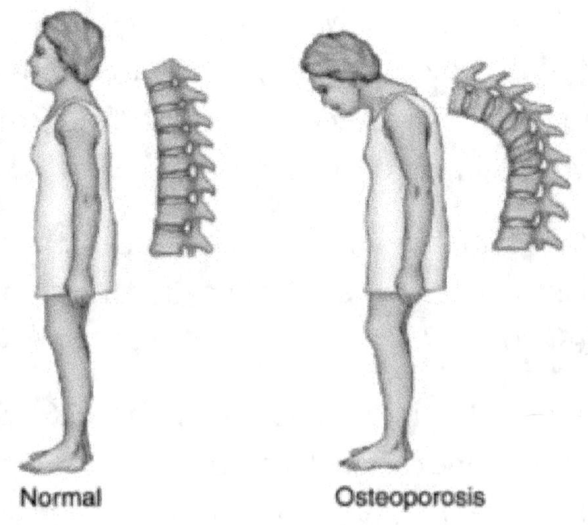

Osteoporosis is a conditions that weakens bones. It makes them fragile – so fragile that there is often more hollow space than bone. I have known people who have coughed and fractured vertebrae.

This condition didn't come on overnight. It developed over years and it is only generally diagnosed when a fracture, after a minor injury, occurs.

---

[3] http://osteocenterny.com/osteoporosis-education/

These fractures generally occur in vertebrae, wrists and hips. However, they are not confined to these bones. A sneeze can cause rib fractures or the partial collapse of a vertebrae.

The Dowager's hump which is characteristic of osteoporosis occurs when bones in the spine become deformed.

Approximately, 3 million people in the UK are affected by osteoporosis. This doesn't take into account those who have osteoporosis but are not aware of the damage inside their body.

There are a number of people who are at risk from osteoporosis. They include:

- Those on steroid therapy as steroids leach calcium from bones. This will include those with asthma, auto immune diseases, among others.
- Those whose diet lacks vitamin D since vitamin D helps bones take up calcium
- Those who don't get out into the sun since the sun provides much of the vitamin D that we require.

- Those with inflammatory bowel disease who have difficulty absorbing nutrients.
- The elderly – as age increases, appetite reduces as does our ability to absorb nutrients from our diet.

This is not a definitive list.

Now much of the pain relief that I recommended for lumbago in the earlier part of the book also applies to osteoporosis and osteoarthritis, but, in addition, we need to add further nutrients to the diet to help build back up strong healthy bone.

As we have seen glycine is a must as it has oestrogen like effects and therefore contributes to building healthy bones but we must also add three other amino acids – proline, hydroxyproline and arginine which are essential components of collagen; collagen is the major protein found in bone and other connective tissue.

Luckily, all the amino acids can be found in gelatin so the first consideration is to take 15mg of gelatin a day. This can be in the form of bone broth, or gelatin incorporated into sweet or savoury dishes, fish head soup. Confectionary, like wine gums, are also made from gelatin but tend to contain a lot of glucose which is not advised for diabetics.

The minerals and vitamins we need to make sure that are incorporated into the diet, in order to avoid bone fragility are:

- Boron
- Magnesium
- Calcium
- Vitamin C
- Vitamin D
- Vitamin K
- zinc

We have already addressed boron so we shall look at the properties of magnesium and calcium next.

Most people already incorporate enough calcium into their diet but give little attention to magnesium. However, lack of magnesium is a major factor in osteoporosis.

Nevertheless, there are different forms of calcium; the calcium that is oft prescribed – calcium carbonate - is not very absorbable and needs an acidic stomach to do so, calcium citrate does not need a highly acidic stomach and so is more suitable for the elderly who tend to have reduced stomach acid.

Magnesium participates in hundreds of biochemical reactions in the body some of which harden bones and teeth. Further, you can have as much calcium in your diet as you like but, without magnesium the absorption and metabolism of calcium will not happen.

Magnesium also stimulates the production of calcitonin. This is a hormone which helps preserve bone. It also regulates another hormone – parathyroid hormone - which prevents the breakdown of bone.

Magnesium is also responsible for converting vitamin D into its active form.

Those who have a poor dietary intake of magnesium are setting themselves up for osteoporosis. Further, those on diuretics will leach magnesium into urine leading to a deficiency in this important mineral. Magnesium also helps to regulate pain.

Foods which contain good amounts of magnesium are green leafy vegetables and nuts.

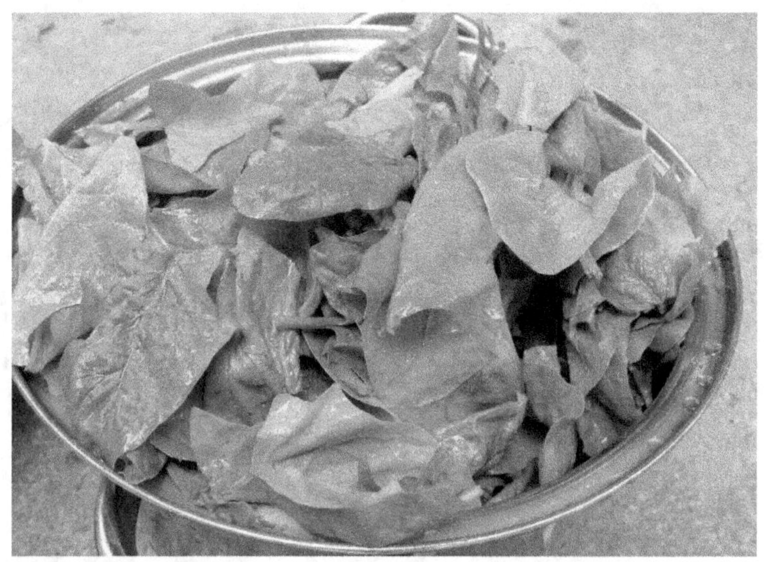

Spinach; a good source of magnesium

Vitamin C

This vitamin is essential in helping form good bone tissue. This is because a large part of bone is formed from collagen. The four major amino acids which build bone are:

- Glycine
- Proline

- Hydroxyproline
- Arginine.

Proline requires vitamin C to convert into Hydroxyproline. Without vitamin C the major building blocks for collagen are not available so hard dense bone cannot be built up.

Please see diagram below

Diagram showing chain of events in forming collagen from glutamic acid.

↓

Glutamic Acid

↓

Proline and vitamin C

↓

Hydroxyproline

↓

+ glycine (from serine) and arginine =

Collagen peptides

Vitamin D

In the 1950's, it was not unusual to be dosed with cod liver oil every day to avoid diseases like rickets which were rife in those days. The practice died off although our diets did not improve. Even if they had, it is near impossible to get enough vitamin D from the diet.

 Most of the vitamin D we have is gleaned from the action of the sun on our skin. This is fine but English summers do not boast a lot of sunlight.

Between October and April, there isn't enough sunlight to penetrate our skin and we don't store enough in the summer months to last us over winter.

We also become less efficient at making our own vitamin D, through the action of sunlight on our skin, as we get older. If this wasn't enough, we have a habit of sloshing sun cream on our skin which effectively prevents the synthesis of vitamin D.

Vitamin D is essential for bone health as it regulates the amount of calcium in the body.

Without enough vitamin D, osteomalacia – soft and weak bones, in adults – and rickets, in children, will occur.

Surprisingly, lack of vitamin D can be responsible for poor hearing since the bones can go soft in the ear, too.

Sources of vitamin D

- Sunlight
- Egg yolk
- Oily fish
- Enriched cereals – check on the packet

Vitamin D is a fat soluble vitamin and requires a little fat to be absorbed.

Vitamin K – vitamin K is an essential nutrient that helps build strong bones. Studies have found that people with higher blood levels of this vitamin have a higher bone density[4] and those with low levels of vitamin K are more likely to have osteoporosis.

---

[4] University of Maryland Medical Center. Vitamin K. http://www.umm.edu/health/medical/altmed/supplement/vitamin-k Last reviewed 7/13/2013. Accessed 12-21-17

We require 90 micrograms of vitamin K daily for women and 120 mcg for men.

Good sources of this are dark green leafy vegetables such as chard and spinach. In matters of preventing osteoporosis, we are looking at two good helpings of this daily.

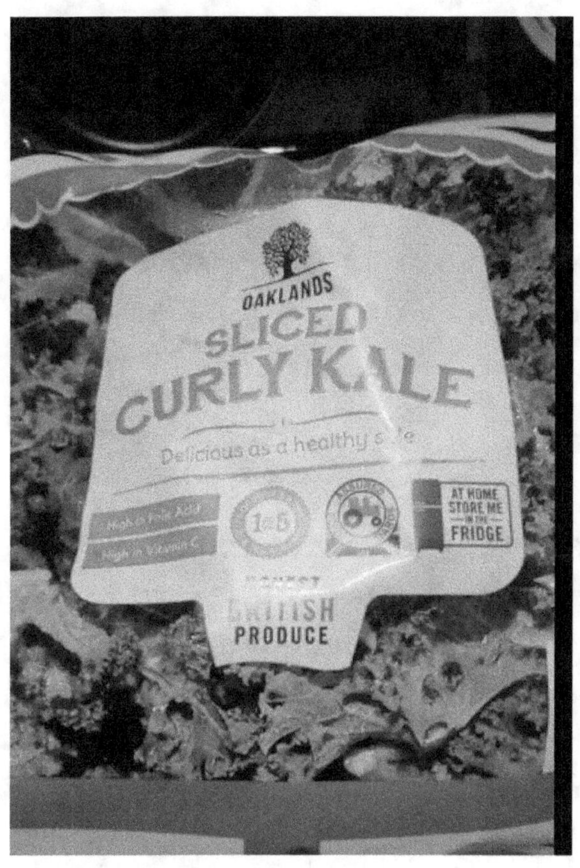

Kale is an excellent source of vitamin K

Like vitamin D, vitamin K is also fat soluble and should be eaten with a little fat to help absorption.

Table showing amount of vitamin K in foods[5]

Food/serving size	Vitamin K µgm
½ cup broccoli	110
½ cup Brussels sprouts	150
½ cup cooked kale	550
½ cup raw kale	274
1 cup raw endive	116
½ cup beet greens	350
½ cup raw collard greens	418
½ cup cooked collard greens	530
½ cup cooked spinach	444
1 cup raw spinach	145
½ cup mustard greens	210
½ cup Swiss chard	287

There are people with various conditions who should monitor their intake of vitamin K as it can inhibit clotting. Therefore, people on warfarin, for example, should seek medical advice if they are considering supplementing with this nutrient.

Therefore, to address problems associated with osteoporosis I would recommend:

---

[5] National Osteoporosis Foundation.
Nutrition. https://www.nof.org/patients/treatment/nutrition/ Assessed 12-26-17

Nutrient	RDA
gelatin	15mg
boron	6mg
Vitamin D	2000 iu's
Vitamin C	500-1000mg
magnesium	500mg
Vitamin K	90 mcg
calcium	1200mg

For cartilage problems associated with osteoporosis add 2mg of manganese.

Manganese (not to be confused with magnesium) is vital for healthy cartilage. It helps in the synthesis of enzymes involved in the synthesis of

Glycosaminoglycan

Collagen (type 2)

Proteoglycan

Found in cartilage

The articular cartilage found at the ends of the bones in a joint which enables smooth movement is particularly high in manganese.

Manganese is found in a wide range of foods including:

Chickpeas

Kidney beans

Lentils

Soybeans

Hazelnuts

Pecans

Whole grains

Shellfish

Leafy green vegetables like chard

The importance of copper

When most people think of osteoporosis the importance of copper in preventing this condition does not come to mind. Certainly, I have never heard of copper and osteoporosis uttered together in the same breath as I have heard with vitamin D and osteoporosis.

 When a copper deficiency occurs then damaged connective tissue cannot be replaced with collagen that makes up the scaffolding of the bone. Copper, simply, is required to prevent osteoporosis.

The recommended daily allowance of copper is 900mcg. However, as a deficiency or excess of copper can have potentially negative effects then supplementation is not recommended unless under medical supervision. Instead, incorporating foods, containing copper, into the diet - where there appears to be a lack of them - is a sensible way forward.

 Incorporating copper containing foods into the diet will begin the process of synthesising the collagen that is required for the scaffolding of connective tissue in bone formation.

Foods which contain good amounts of copper include:

- Liver and other organ meats
- Oysters
- Dark chocolate
- Spirulina
- Nuts and seeds
- Lobster
- Leafy greens
- Shitake mushrooms

Although liver is an excellent source of copper, three ounces of liver provides over 1,000% of the recommended daily allowance of copper. In cases of known deficiency where osteoporosis has been diagnosed, a portion of liver, once or twice a week, will not be frowned upon especially as it contains vitamin D which is also required for strong bones.

Tests for copper deficiency are available through your GP.

Copper deficiency is especially to be found in the elderly as the ability to absorb nutrients falters with age. Further, a reduction in appetite that accompanies older age means that a deficiency of copper is more likely to occur, anyway.

It is not surprising that twenty percent of Caucasian women age 50 or over are estimated to have osteoporosis.

Other signs of copper deficiency include:

- Weakness and fatigue
- Sensitivity to cold
- Frequently getting sick
- Difficulty in retaining information
- Pale skin
- Premature greying
- Difficulties with walking – wide, waddling gait
- Vision and colour loss
- Peripheral neuropathy

Some people buy copper bracelets to reduce the inflammatory processes that cause pain in many arthritic conditions. Do they work? Can copper penetrate the skin? For years many people thought that any pain reduction experienced was due to the placebo effect. However, studies have shown that trace amounts of copper do penetrate the skin. Perhaps enough, arguably, to replace that lost through poor absorption or poor diet, in later years.

copper bracelets do appear to release particles of copper which penetrate the skin and assist in lowering inflammation.

We have now covered pain relief for back problems and nutrients which will help build healthy bones and connective tissue.

All conditions have slightly different nutrient requirements and back pain is no different. The building and remodelling of bone and cartilage takes slightly longer but it will happen provided it is afforded the correct building blocks to do so.

Finally, bone and cartilage becomes denser during the pounding which is undertaken during walking and weight bearing exercise so this should not be neglected. Articular cartilage is avascular – it does not have a blood supply. Nutrients must be absorbed into the cartilage so a regular and adequate supply must be available for delivery to the chondrocytes. The alternating compression and decompression that occurs during exercise assists in the delivery of the nutrients to the chondrocytes.

 Exercise also helps to keep muscles in trim so that injury is less likely to occur. Exercise such as gardening, a stroll to the shop and housework are effective.

Can we be confident that disc pain can alleviated?

An article by Ressel[6] has found clinical and experimental evidence that cartilage damaged by trauma, injury or movement disorders can be healed and regenerated. He goes on to say that 'the degree of repair and regeneration of intervertebral discs is greatly dependent on the character of the extracellular 'scaffold' (see section on copper), the available nutrition, the age and biomechanical state of the diskal material.'

This raises the possibility that the reversal of osteoarthritic changes is within our grasp. Ressel notes further that

The time interval necessary for improvement to manifest varied from as little as two months to over seven years, and was dependent on the

---

[6] Ressel OJ. Disk regeneration: reversibility is possible in spinal osteoarthritis. ICA International Review of Chiropractic March/April 1989;39-61.

degree of compliance to a multifaceted regime and the extent of the degeneration, among other things.'

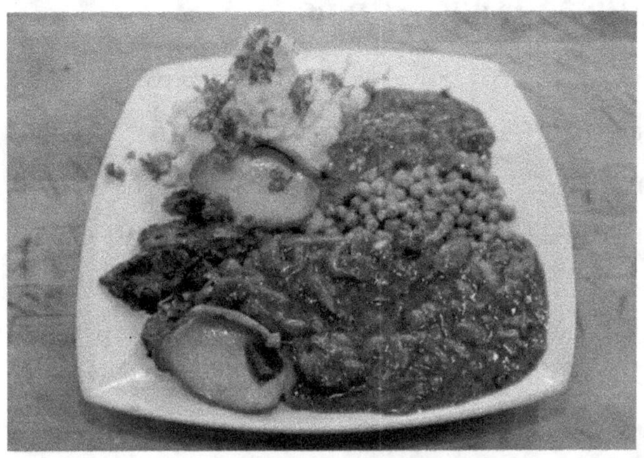

A meal of liver and onions weekly does much to ameliorate joint and bone problems associated with older age

You are probably going to say, 'Well, what about glucosamine and chondroitin sulphate. These are popular supplements. Are they any good? It is to these that we will now turn our attention.

Chondroitin and Glucosamine

Chondroitin sulphate and glucosamine are popular over the counter supplements that are used to treat pain and loss of function found in osteoarthritis. Some people swear by these supplements and others don't. This doesn't present a mystery. When we look at any disorder such as osteoarthritis, there are a number of nutritional deficiencies that can contribute to the disease process and any one deficiency can tip the status quo into an inflammatory disease. Therefore, if any one individual has arthritis due to a vitamin D deficiency then no amount of glucosamine will meet the body's need for this vitamin. However, if glucosamine or chondroitin is contributing to the problem then these need to be included – or increased – in the diet.

Investigating the causes of disease takes time but it is a necessary task.

Chondroitin is a major component of cartilage that is made in the body. It helps the cartilage retain water providing a cushioning effect between the ends of bone. It is reported to have mild pain relieving effects which take some time to be felt. It may be useful as an adjunctive medicine.

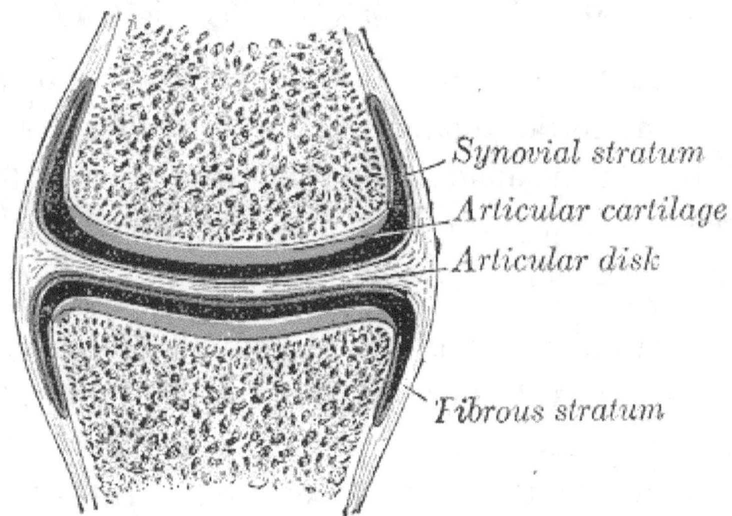

Articular cartilage is full of chondroitin so long slow cooking of bones to make bone broth which was common practise in the 1950's made a valuable broth for joint health

As we age we become less adept at synthesising substances such as chondroitin. It is not surprising that osteoarthritis occurs as we age and are less able to synthesise nutrients or absorb them from our diet.

Supplemental chondroitin is made from the cartilage of animals. Cartilage contains a great deal of cooked collagen, known as gelatin.

Glucosamine is a natural substance found in healthy cartilage although the majority is to be found in the fluid around joints. It appears to help cartilage regenerate and has anti-inflammatory properties.

Glucosamine may provide some relief for those with osteoarthritis of the hip, knee and spine. It has not been reported to have any side effects and may be used for mild pain relief instead of NSAID's which do have a number of negative side effects.

Some people have argued that glucosamine pain relieving effects are simply due to the placebo effect. However, the first phase of the

GALT study (Glucosamine/Chondroitin Arthritis Intervention Trial) did find that a combination of both substances showed significant pain relief in those with moderate to severe pain in knee osteoarthritis. However, these results were not replicated in those with mild knee pain.

Bone broth contains chondroitin and glucosamine and hyaluronic acid. These are all substances that help to reduce inflammation and consequently, joint pain.

Hyaluronic acid

Joints need to be well lubricated in order to work effectively. Synovial fluid provides the 'oil' for joints, allowing the bones to glide over each other. Synovial fluid contains a substance known as hyaluronic acid but in people with osteoarthritis this substance breaks down. The lack of hyaluronic acid increases joint pain and stiffness.

Hyaluronic acid is given into the joint by injection and appears to have significant effects in many – but not all – people who have received this form of treatment.

Hyaluronic acid is a useful treatment option for patients who cannot tolerate NSAID's. NSAID's have potentially unwanted side effects and should be avoided, if possible. NSAID's, for example, can cause stomach bleeding or kidney problems in susceptible people.

A review of the effectiveness of hyaluronic acid was undertaken by Nicholas Bellamy, MD, and his team at the University of Queensland in Brisbane, in 2006. In total, 76 studies were reviewed that had examined the effect of hyaluronic acid for treating knee osteoarthritis. The review found that pain levels were reduced by 28-54 percent for the average patient who received injections into the knee. This was in line with the amount of pain reduction found in patients who took NSAID's.

It was also found that hyaluronic acid improved the ability to move about and perform daily activities by 9-32%.

As I have already stated, hyaluronic acid production diminishes as you age. It can be applied topically but it can't reach the deepest layers of skin. However, DMSO, a solvent with powerful penetrating properties and anti-inflammatory properties can be used to help hyaluronic acid to penetrate further into the tissues.

However, the best way to increase levels of hyaluronic acid is simply by increasing foods that contain this substance or foods that help increase hyaluronic acid synthesis. As usual bone broth provides ample amounts provided it is simmered slowly for many hours to help leach the goodness out.

Foods that help increase oestrogen has the potential to increase the production of hyaluronic acid. Such foods include:

- Soy based products

- Tempeh
- Tofu
- Edamame beans

Citrus fruits contain a substance call naringenin. This helps to prevent the breakdown of hyaluronic acid in the body. In addition to citrus fruits, tomatoes and bananas also contain naringenin.

The production of hyaluronic acid is also increased by the addition of starchy root vegetables to the diet. These foods include:

- Potatoes
- Sweet potatoes
- Jerusalem artichoke

Leafy greens contain magnesium. Magnesium is required to help with hyaluronic acid in the body. As people age they are more likely to be placed on diuretics which have the undesirable effect of removing magnesium from the body. Magnesium has over 300 functions in the body so its impact, when deficient, is enormous. Everybody should get into the habit of eating a portion of green leafy vegetables every day. Other foods that contain good amounts of magnesium are nuts and seeds.

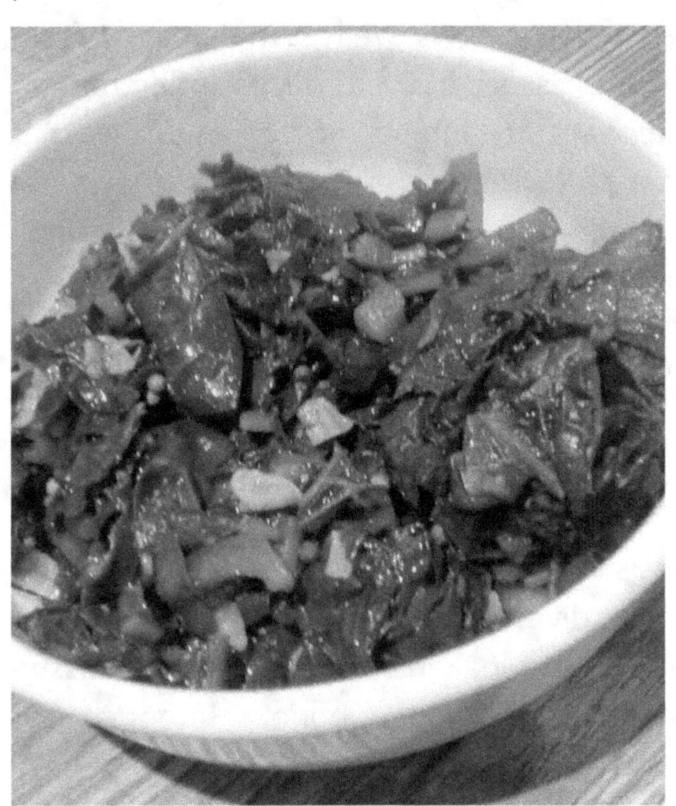

Chard with red pepper – full of magnesium!

Methylsulfonylmethane (MSM)

MSM is an organic sulphur compound that occurs naturally in many fruits, vegetables and grains especially broccoli, Brussels sprouts, garlic and onion. It is needed to help form connective tissue. As well as helping to form connective tissue, MSM reduces inflammation and appears to inhibit nerve impulses that transmit pain. Therefore, MSM would be useful for treating pain like sciatica and even migraine and shingles.

MSM comes in a variety of forms including, powder, tablets and incorporated into cream for topical use.

You have probably gathered by now that the synthesis of connective tissue is complex and requires a diverse diet; removal or deficiency of any nutrient weakens the connective tissue whether that is cartilage, bone, tendon, skin or ligament.

When tissue is not synthesised properly then injury, pain, stiffness and inflammation is the result.

Not all the damage can be seen immediately, osteoporosis is silent for the most part until someone tries to turn over in bed and finds that their vertebrae has fractured somewhere.

It's simply not worth getting to that point; while most conditions are reversible, the loss of two inches in height with accompanying pain is not worth it.

There are few side effects with MSM but these include stomach upset or diarrhoea.

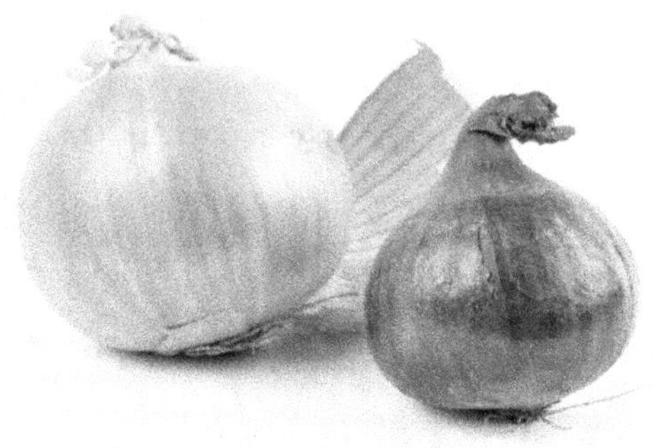

Onions contain MSM and help protect bones by its involvement in the synthesis of connective tissue. MSM also help inhibit nerve impulses that transfer pain. They also contain boron which is needed to help reduce inflammation and help 'harden' bones.

MSM is safe, according to the Food and Drug Administration if given in no larger doses than 4000mg (4g)

In energy bars it is found in amounts of up to 30,000mg per kg daily; this equates to 30g daily if just one energy bar containing this amount is eaten.

To give you an idea of the amount of sulphur in animal protein per 100g:

Turkey 910mg

Chicken breast 900mg

Pork 880 mg

Liver 850mg

 Beef 740mg

The good news is that supplementation of 1200mg was effective in alleviating pain although the full effect was not felt for up to 12 weeks.

Onions have differing amounts of sulphur

Red onions = 50mg per 100g of onion

Brown onions = 9.3 mg per 100g of onion

Spring onion = 23.6 mg per 100g of onion

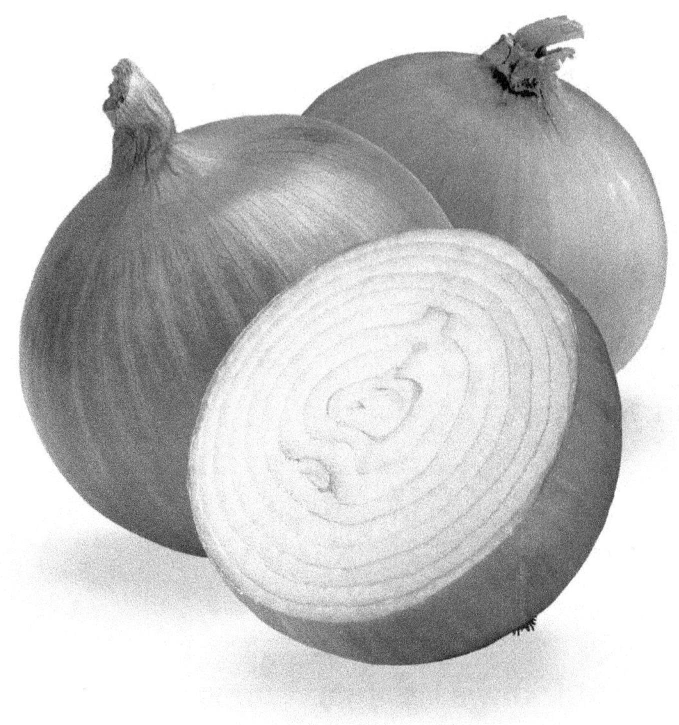

Red onions have higher amounts of sulphur than brown or spring onions

Chronic pain versus acute pain

Acute pain is what we feel at the time of injury whether that is due to too much gardening or wrenching the back unnaturally when attempting to lift a box.

When injury strikes then the muscles normally go into spasm immediately to provide a rigid scaffold to prevent further injury. This scaffold of muscle is so effective that it can prevent any movement

Here is a little anecdote of when I happened to have finished private tuition, my pupil had departed and I was clearing up the pencils and paper. We had used some equipment to illustrate the lesson and it was at the far side of the table so I leaned over.....

My back went into spasm and I could not move from the position that I was in. Bemused my husband fetched me the phone so that I could ring the GP who helpfully suggested that I turn up at the surgery at 2pm, some 3 hours later.

Clearly, I had not conveyed the urgency of the situation to him in a way that enhanced his understanding.

I tried again and this time he realised the urgency of the situation and said he would write a prescription out for Baclofen if my husband could collect it. He did.

The Baclofen, an oft prescribed anti-spasmodic did help enough for me to manage to rise from leaning over the table but, for long enough, I hobbled with small irregular steps. I found getting into bed, off a chair, dressing, in fact most activities of daily living just about impossible.

I wondered how most people without a relative to support them would manage. Bad backs are not classed as urgent although they certainly disrupt living with a vengeance.

 The pain can be debilitating and rarely responds to the prescriptions that are dished out and which you must try for six weeks before a referral to a physiotherapist can be made.

As everyone knows, even when a referral is made that is just the beginning of a long wait before the actual appointment.

Bad backs are no respecter of persons. Sometimes they just 'go' for no apparent reason at all as happened to me once when I was opening a drawer and my back just 'went.' It was half an hour before I could inch round to move across the floor in slow painstaking steps.

For some people with connective tissue disorders bad backs and joint problems are intimately connected to this condition. Lax tissue allows over extension of the joint so that walking on a pebble can result in the joint not able to support the change resulting in a loss of balance and possible falls.

Chronic pain is any pain that continues beyond twelve weeks. It is pathological – disease based – pain because the body is designed to heal; when it does not, in the expected time for that particular body tissue, then it requires further investigation.

Most conditions will then have 'itis' tagged onto them which is simply a reference to inflammation.

'Itis' conditions tend to become rife the older we get. The body does not appear to be able to heal the same although, in most cases, this is entirely due to the lack of nutritional intake whether it be due to poorer absorption of what would have once been adequate nutrition.

More than once have my husband and I bemoaned that we do not have the same appetite as we once had.

In order to overcome that, smaller but more nutritionally dense foods have to be eaten. Supplementation may need to be considered especially in relation to vitamin D.

The non- inflammatory animal fats should be chosen over and above inflammatory seed oils.

Never let anyone tell you that pain is part and parcel of the ageing process and that nothing can be done apart from taking prescription medications.

This is simply not true; pain alerts us to something that needs fixing. Prescription medications generally mask the symptoms but do nothing to rectify the underlying cause.

When a medic informs you that nothing can be done then they are simply saying within their branch of medicine or within the limits of their source of funding. Try an osteopath or a medical nutritionist and the answer will probably be different. Nutritional medicine often provides the answer when conventional medicine has failed to.

Let's face it, the body runs on vitamins and minerals, on macromolecules like fats, proteins and carbohydrates. It does not run on medication but so many people are convinced that is the way to health.

We must not forget that rest and exercise are essential too since the former is when the body begins to repair itself.

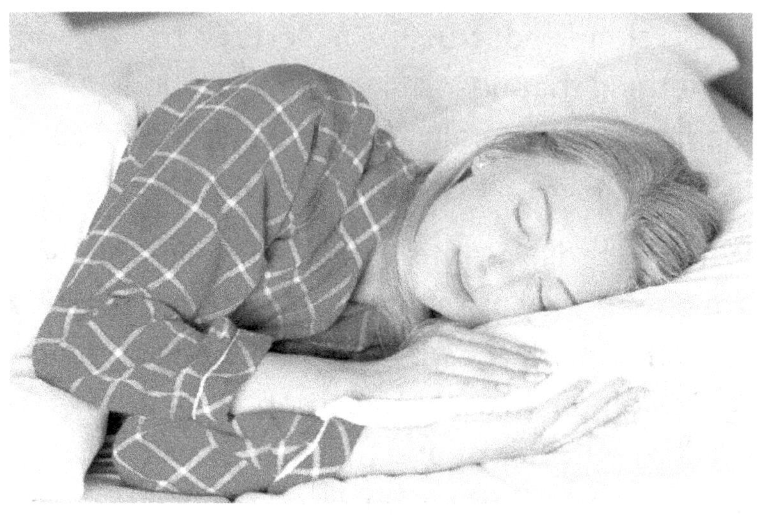

Sleep is restorative

Postural problems

On a less dramatic note, all sorts of postural problems affecting the back start from the position of weak ankles. Many people appear to suffer from weak ankles with ankle pronation – inward rolling of the foot – high on the list of factors which can be a risk for bad backs.

Ankle pronation can be due to many reasons including:

 A genetic link where there is a familial history of low arches and flat feet.

Injuries; especially in those who are active in sports

 Low muscle tone

Pregnancy and/or obesity can stretch ligaments

Unsupportive shoes can also be a risk for over-pronation

There are also numerous health conditions which are a risk factor for over pronation and these include:

Arthritis

Cerebral palsy

Muscular dystrophy

Spinal bifida

Diabetes

The ageing process

The difficulty with over pronation is that the problem just does not affect the ankles; it has a knock on effect, affecting knees, hips and spine.

It is more or less certain that if the sole of the foot suffers pain, that this pathological mechanical state will transmit upwards.

That sciatica which is the bane of your life may well be due to the weak ankles you have inherited from your mother's or father's side.

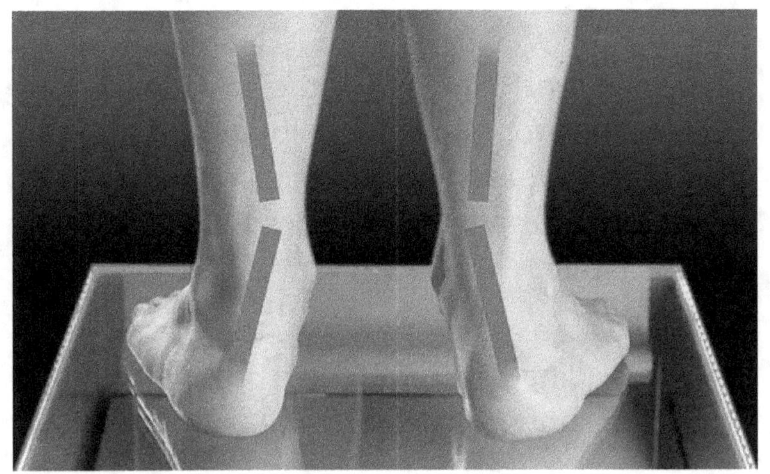

Over-pronation of the feet.

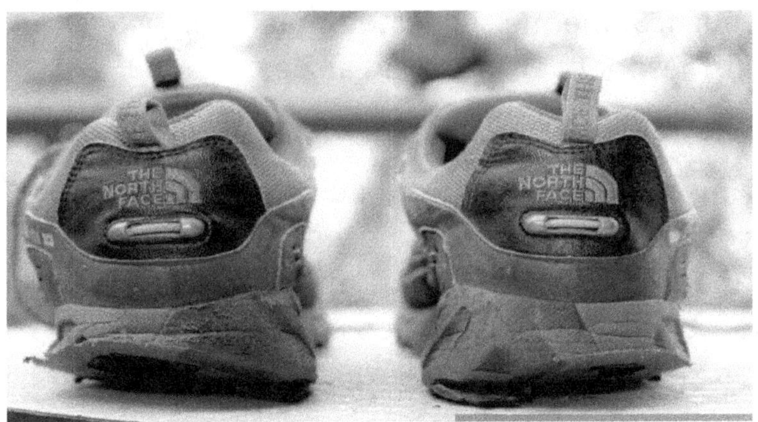

Over-pronation of the foot can affect one foot more than the other leading to an imbalance which may mean that sciatica only ever occurs on one side of the body.

It is always worth looking at the soles of the shoes to look for uneven distribution of the soles of the shoes. People appear to take more notice of the tread of their tyres than their feet, unfortunately.

It is also worth asking someone to take a photo of you standing barefoot to see how well your ankles are supporting the rest of your body.

One of my relatives had intractable knee pain. He had investigations which did not reveal much. Someone suggested that he buy some insoles for over pronated ankles.

They did the trick!

However, if my relative had continued without correcting his posture, he would have undoubtedly gone on to suffer from hip or back problems. The spine needs to be aligned properly otherwise will cause untold pain and disability.

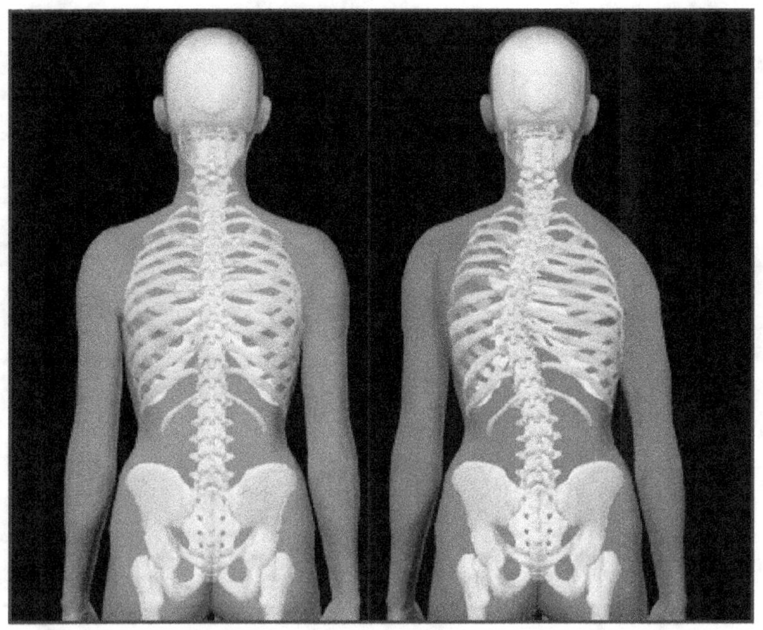

Contrast the above two pictures and begin to understand the problems caused by a misaligned spine.

Apart from insoles which can help correct over pronation, weak ankles will benefit from an ankle support to prevent overstretching of the joints. There is a huge range of ankle supports to choose from; some cost little and are little more than a glorified band of wide elastic.

Some are much more expensive encasing the leg as well as ankle. Often they will have rigid side panels which provide even further support so that balance is more likely to be maintained.

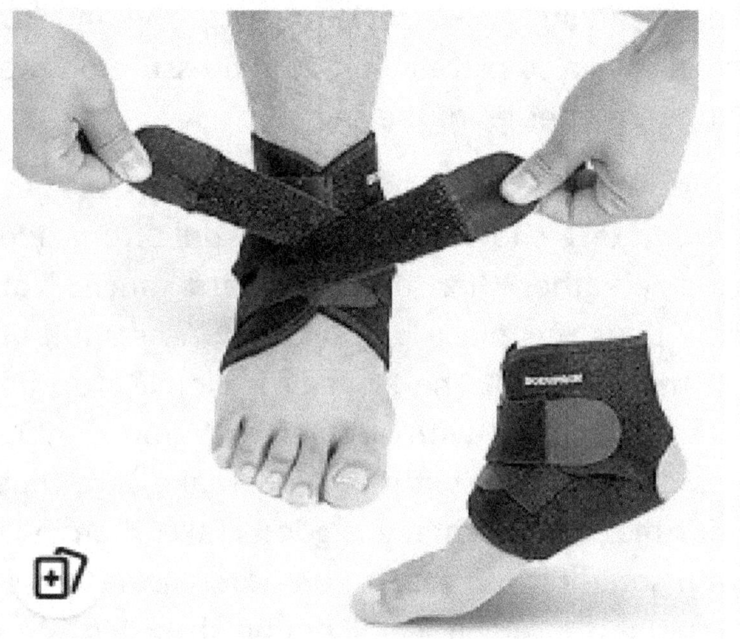

Ankle braces come in different shapes and sizes. If you are not sure what you need then it is worth making an appointment with a podiatrist.

Some that come with the more rigid side panels have been known to rub on the ankle bone especially if it is more prominent so it is wise to try - or at least consider – a number before settling on one.

The waddling gait associated with a vitamin D deficiency also places unnatural pressure on the wonderful design of the spine.

When elderly are deficient in vitamin D they tend to take shorter steps and waddle from side to side rather than move forward much. Not only does this place pressure on the spine but on the hips too. The remedy is simple, top up vitamin D levels with supplements about 4000 iu's daily on days without sun. Make sure that your magnesium intake is good. Take vitamin D with some fat for absorption otherwise there is no point in taking it, it will not be absorbed.

This brings me to the point about the foolishness of prescribing elderly the calcium cum vitamin D supplements. My aunt used to be prescribed them; one to be taken with a glass of water. Where the fat for absorption or magnesium to enhance activation of vitamin D was in this prescription, I do not know. It really was not helpful.

There are many conditions that I have not mentioned such as:

Ankylosing spondylitis

Psoriatic arthritis

Arachnoiditis

Discitis

Sacroilitis

But they really do not need a separate chapter all to themselves; they are all 'itis' conditions; inflammatory conditions which will respond well to the nutritional medicine mentioned in this book. They have one underlying cause which is inflammation, the name of the condition merely describes where the inflammation is and what it affects.

Stiffness and pain is part of the inflammatory process.

Inflammation will manifest itself if there is injury or infection present.

Infection can be treated with antibiotics or high dose vitamin C (between 3g-6g is suitable for infection).

If there is a time when known injury occurred then healing needs to take place; meanwhile, there is plenty of choice of nutritional medicine to help alleviate the pain while healing is ongoing.

Spasms are dealt with by pushing a small blunt object into the centre of the spasm until it releases.

Back belts are useful for providing support; it's always useful to have one in just in case.

If the injury comes on slowly then it is likely to be mechanical in nature due to poor posture such as that found due to excessive ankle pronation. This needs correcting. A good podiatrist is worth their weight in gold and can save hours of pain and disability using their professional skills.

The orthotics department, often a small department tucked away at the back of a hospital somewhere, is one of those departments that is never really appreciated until you have need to use their services.

Their skills make the difference between being unable to participate in mainstream life and becoming a full member of such.

After a fracture in my left foot, which went undiagnosed for over 5 months in spite of my repeated complaints of persistent pain, I suffered from drop foot due to the weakened muscles (I had been unable to walk for 5 months). The drop foot resulted in repeated falls with all the inconvenience of that.

Eventually, unable to go out, I was referred to orthotics who provided a splint which kept my foot in the correct position. In minutes I was able to walk properly and without fear of falling.

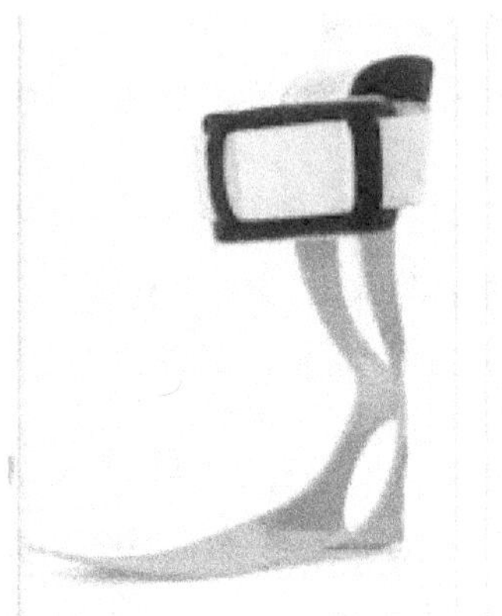

Splints like the above are often prescribed by orthotics departments to enable those who would not be able to get around safely without them

Other clues which suggest that the body is not properly aligned are other conditions that affect the feet such as:

Corns

Plantar fasciitis

Bunions and similar

callous

They may appear so far removed from the back that the connection between them, posture and back problems may not be obvious.

Another thing to watch out for is recurring sprains and strains; all indicators of future joint and back problems.

Nip them in the bud.

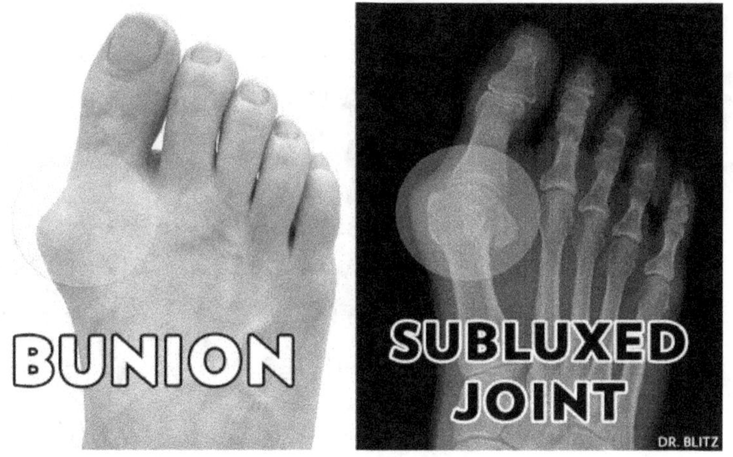

Bunions; indicators of mechanical problems which may impact joint further up the body at some point.

Bulging Discs

One mechanical problem that occurs often is the phenomenon of bulging spinal discs. It is more likely to occur as age progresses and occurs due to:

Loss of fluid so that the discs dry out

Lose their flexibility

The outer layer of the disc is made from cartilage and this protects, and encases, the inner gel like substance within the disc.

As ageing progresses, whether this be due to some nutrient deficiency or not, the outer layer thins so that it does not hold the gel like substance well. This can bulge out.

Now lots of people from their 40's onwards will have some form of bulging disc and most do not cause symptoms. It is more likely to be symptomatic if the bulging disc is pressing on a nerve.

Sometimes the inner gel part of the disc ruptures and bulges through the outer layer. This is then

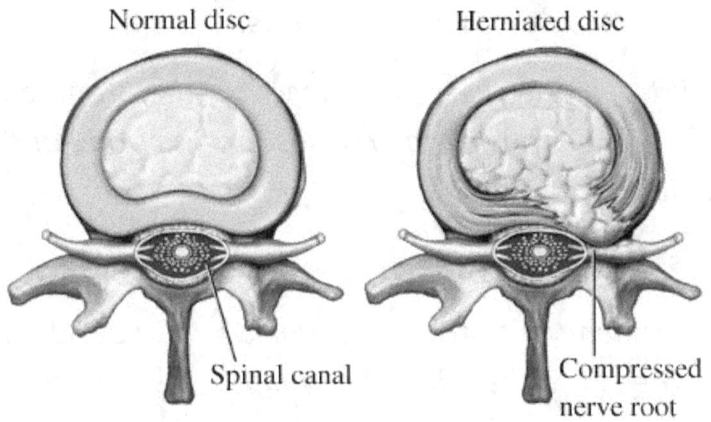

Top views of vertebrae

referred to as a herniated disc and can cause a number of symptoms such as:

Numbness and tingling in the lower limbs

Weakness in the lower limbs

Pain

Most of the time a herniated disc is due to fall injuries or repetitive movements.

Not following the rules when lifting heavy items can also result in herniated discs.

To lift weight, keep as close to the item as possible. Keep the elbows close to the body and the back straight.

The stomach muscles should be tightened.

Do not bend over from the waist but by bending the knees and keeping the weight close, draw it up.

Bending over or twisting is almost guaranteed to injure the back.

Herniated discs are painful and take from 4-6 weeks to heal. It is recommended that people remain active although this is difficult due to the pain, stiffness and muscle spasm that occurs.

The stiffness is due to inflammatory chemicals which cause leaky blood vessels and fluid entering cellular spaces. High dose vitamin C does address inflammation very well but you will probably not get enough in the recommended 5 a day or even 10 a day.

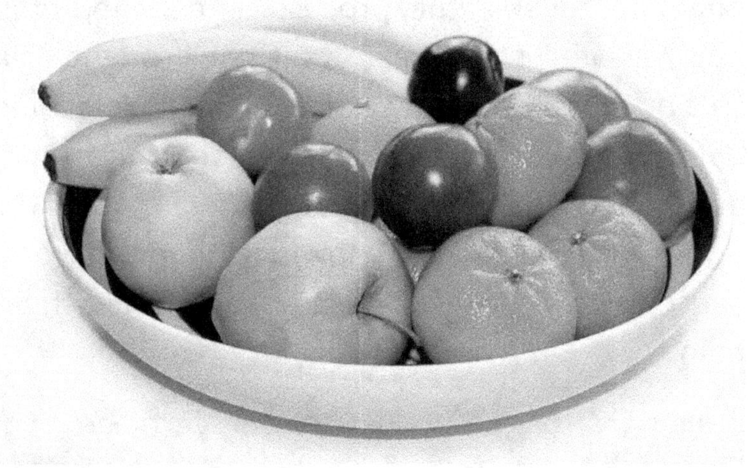

Fruit contains vitamin C which helps reduce inflammation but fruit probably does not contain enough vitamin C to make a great deal of difference to a back injury. Supplementation will be required.

However, the pain does respond to the nutrients I have mentioned and this enables activity to be undertaken although sudden movements will not be appreciated. Back belts really do help in this respect and they provide warmth which helps soothe muscle spasms.

This appears to be a good place to stop. We now have enough knowledge to be able to begin to reverse the process of degeneration and relieve the back pain that has brought you to buy this book in the first place. Alleviating pain involves investigating the root cause and addressing it. Each person's journey is unique but in the process of investigating the root cause of pain, they will be taking control of their pain

Building stronger bones, denser cartilage and healthier tendons and ligaments and, in the process, eliminating pain starts as soon as the above is put into practice.

Useful Information

Cartilage is made up of four substances:

- Collagen
- Proteoglycans
- Water
- chondrocytes

Collagen is primarily made up of these main amino acids

- glycine
- proline
- hydroxyproline
- arginine

Adequate vitamin C is required to convert proline to Hydroxyproline.

<u>A lack of proline in the diet can be responsible for strains and tears in soft tissue and a poor rate of healing.</u> Proline also helps to prevent arteriosclerosis – hardening of the arteries – and assists in balancing blood pressure levels.

Further, proline also helps the body break down protein from worn out cells in the body. The end result of this degradation is then used to create new healthy cells.

 Proline is also required to form hydroxyproline.

Hydroxyproline is another amino acid which is a major component of the protein, collagen.

Good sources of proline are: egg yolks, grass fed meats, organ meats – for example, liver and kidney, bone broth and gelatin. Many of these simply do not form part of our diet anymore in any great amount.

This inadequacy leaves us vulnerable to back injury.

Good sources of proline are:

Chicken with the skin left on

Pork rinds

Any animal protein, bone broth, gelatine and eggs

Soy

Nuts

Legumes

Kidney beans

Mushrooms

Peanuts

cabbage

<u>Diagram showing chain of events in forming collagen from glutamic acid.</u>

Glutamic Acid

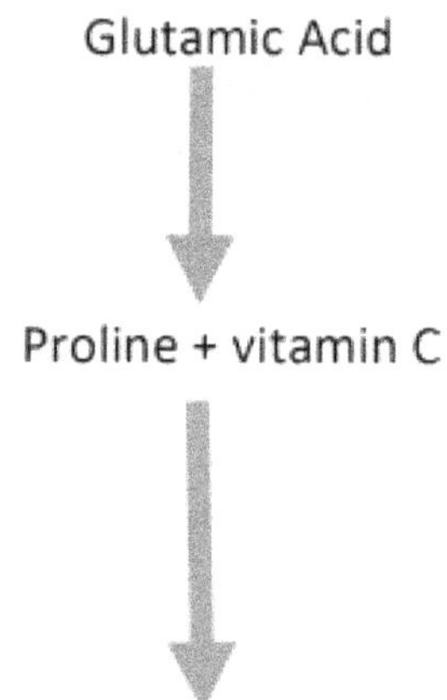

Proline + vitamin C

hydroxyproline + glycine (from serine) and arginine

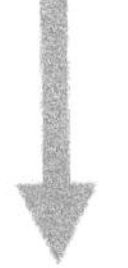

Collagen peptides

What happens in inflammation?

We talk about inflammation a lot. We recognise inflammation as it causes pain, stiffness, swelling and redness but what is happening underneath the surface that contributes to this?

Inflammation is a property of the defence system of the host which protects it from infection and injury. It brings about the means to destroy pathogens but also helps in tissue repair.

Many immune system cells interact with each other to achieve this outcome against the battle raging in the body; it is not dissimilar to the diverse troops engaged in war, all working alongside each other to achieve a successful outcome.

The communication which takes place during this planned assault is undertaken by a number of chemicals known generally as chemokines or cytokines.

It is all these cells and chemicals that that produce the signs of inflammation: heat, redness, pain, swelling and loss of function.

This response is well-regulated so it doesn't get out of hand. It is self-limiting and the activation of mechanisms of negative feedback enable this.

The immune response is exquisite and involves:

The shedding of receptors for inflammatory mediators which lie on the surface of cells. Receptors are tiny and grab onto specific substances. Thus receptors for inflammatory mediator's grab hold of these if they are needed to coordinate an inflammatory defence. Conversely, when inflammation needs to be resolved then the cell sheds these receptors. Other well-known receptors are the vitamin D receptor which is found in every cell and tissue of the body and thus, emphasising the importance of sufficient vitamin D for overall health.

When the usual regulatory processed break down then excessive inflammation or chronic inflammation can cause ongoing and deterioration damage to tissues. This is then known as 'disease.'

The acute inflammation required for destruction of pathogens and repair of damaged tissues turns into chronic inflammation. There is a shift in the type of cells found at sites of inflammation. While healing continues it does so alongside other cells still destroying tissue. Which will win?

Of course, if the destructive forces of the immune system hold the upper hand then the tissue will be destroyed slowly accompanied by increasing pain, loss of function, swelling, stiffness. It is not always recognised immediately until you realise that the nagging ache means you can't walk as far to the shops or that your knee appears to be swollen and you cannot climb steps as easily. It may come and go for any meal eaten may contain nutrients which apply brakes to the destructive inflammatory forces or conversely, fuel them. This is how powerful nutritional medicine is.

Thank you for purchasing this book.

Every time a book is purchased, a donation is made to one of the charities I am currently supporting. These can be found on the author's website.

https://www.amazon.co.uk/-/e/B07BPQZ5CD